Partnerships

Practice

The GP's guide to getting it right first time

PETRE JONES

GENERAL PRACTITIONER AND COURSE
ORGANISER, NEWHAM, EAST LONDON

FOREWORD BY
MIKE PRINGLE

RADCLIFFE MEDICAL PRESS

Radcliffe Medical Press Ltd
18 Marcham Road, Abingdon, Oxon OX14 1AA

British Library Cataloguing in Publication Data

A catalogue record for this book is available from the British Library.

ISBN 1 85775 359 3

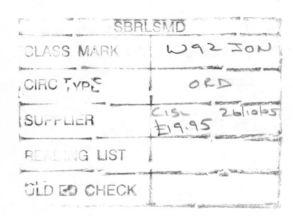
Typeset by Acorn Bookwork, Salisbury, Wiltshire
Printed and bound by Biddles Ltd, Guildford and King's Lynn

Contents

Foreword   v
Introduction   vii

1 Core values and the practice ideals   **1**
   Key moral and professional stances   1
   The stereotypes and self-labelled identity:
      the practice culture   3
   Training practice status   5
   Primary Care Group (PCG) involvement   6

2 The partnership dynamic   **7**
   Team roles   7
   Number of partners   9
   Dynamics between partners   12
   Joint responsibility for decisions   16
   How will formal decisions be made?   17
   Practice manager or practice administrator?   18
   Attitudes to part-time or job-share   20
   Assistantships   21
   'Salaried partners'   22
   Patients and personal lists   23
   Mutual assessment periods and progression to parity   24
   Restrictive covenants on leaving   25
   Compulsory expulsion   25

3 Owning or leasing the premises   **27**
   Own (and control) the premises   27

Lease   29
Rent   30

4 Financial issues   **31**
Pooling income   31
Attitudes to outside work   32
Pooling expenses   34
Partnership shares   34
Showing accounts to the interviewee   36
Banking policy and accounts   37
Private patients   38

5 How hard do you want to work?   **41**
Workload   41
Number of sessions   43
Administrative work   44
Leave   44
Out-of-hours work   46

6 Working policies   **49**
Clinical governance within the practice   49
Professional education   50
Clinical policies   50
Practice area   51
In-hours emergency policy   51

7 Final thought   **53**

Appendix: Sources of income and expense   **55**

Index   **57**

Foreword

For most general practitioner principals, choosing their practice is their second biggest decision after choosing their life partner. For many, their practice is a source of succour and support, of friendship and a fulfilled working life. For others, their dysfunctional practice causes stress, unhappiness and even depression. Practice splits are every bit as unpleasant as a divorce.

And yet we tend to decide to enter into a period of mutual assessment on minimal acquaintance. Once in a practice, albeit 'on approval', it can be difficult and expensive to pull out. Wishful thinking leads to hopes that things will get better, that relationships will improve with time.

We all have personal aspirations and expectations from our professional lives. Finding the right team in which all the partners and other team members – increasingly, the practice manager is a key 'partner' – can maximise their potential without inhibiting others, is a formidable task. Some practice characteristics can be objectively determined early on: the numbers and sexes of partners; the list size; the practice building and facilities; staffing levels; involvement in teaching, training or research. Some can be sought: attitudes to continuity of care; access for patients; prevention; home visiting, and so on can help an applicant to understand the value system of the practice. Personalities and relationships are the most difficult to pin down and these are where many partnerships experience real problems.

This excellent short book analyses these issues and offers sensible practical advice, backed up by case studies. Every doctor considering their second biggest decision should ensure they read this book and digest its wisdom.

Professor Mike Pringle
Chairman of Council, Royal College of General Practitioners
Professor of General Practice, Nottingham
June 1999

Introduction

There are many approaches to running a partnership, and no two partnerships will function in quite the same way. This is one of the greatest joys of general practice, but it can also be the general practitioner's greatest headache.

This book has been written to help people who are looking around at different sorts of practice, to get the feel of the variety of different ways in which a practice might run, and help with picking through the minefield of finding a practice that is suitable. Issues covered include legal and financial considerations for partnership deeds, interaction between and core values of partners, and some key policy issues that may cause conflict. It was first written for the Newham General Practitioner Vocational Training Scheme residential course in 1999, as a resource for the main exercise on partnership choices, but there is no reason why it should not also be used 'in real life'. Essentially, this is a list of thoughts and ideas to prompt you to think, and tries not to dictate right or wrong ways of doing things. This is for you to decide after looking at the evidence and considering your own personal situation. In the end you must make your own choice.

The relationship between partners is governed by the partnership deed, which is an important legal document negotiated and agreed between partners with the help of lawyers. The deed may take many forms but there are some areas it will certainly cover, which are included in this guide. Without a deed, the practice is laid wide open to conflict, and would be governed by the out-of-date and inadequate terms of the Partnership Act of 1890, which offers very little security to anyone.

Less formal aspects of the relationship between partners are also important. Whether you can trust and work with these people, and have common values and objectives in the practice will make or break a partnership and therefore the practice, and these areas are also touched upon.

Partnerships, like marriages, can be very supportive, helping partners through difficulties and being a source of strength and encouragement, as well as enjoyment. On the other hand, a dysfunctional partnership can be dreadful, and can paralyse a practice and make partners miserable. There are still too many stories of 'partners' being exploited. While forming partnerships is a tricky process, breaking partnerships is both difficult and expensive, so the key message is to think carefully about what you want and why, and look carefully at any practice you might consider joining. *It is wise to keep a written log of meetings with prospective practices, so that you have a current record of who promised what to whom, and keep this log until you are well established in a practice with a signed partnership deed.* This makes you clear about what is on offer, and, should it all go wrong will form an invaluable record for a lawyer to work from.

At various points in the guide I have put in non-judgemental value rating scales (NJVRS), invented by Roger Neighbour (*The Inner Apprentice* (1992) Kluwer). In these you will see a visual analogue scale set between two statements that represent the tenable but extreme ends of the spectrum of views on a given issue. Neither end is right nor wrong. You can mark on the scale where you feel you would stand on the issue, and this gives an idea of your own core values. These are discussion starters only, not formal personal moral value rating scales, but may help you to relate the guide to your own views

I have also laced the text with a few examples of partnership life. These are all fictional, but some of the insights contained in some of the examples have come from my own practice. I am grateful to my partners for allowing me to do this. The rest are an amalgamation of various bits and pieces that have lodged themselves in my psyche. None of the examples is intended to refer to any other

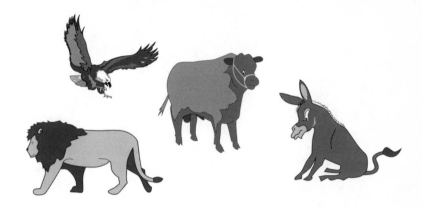

The team?

practice, but are illustrations only. So, if you recognise yourself it could be that you have been absorbed anonymously into my complex delusional system, or it could be that I have tried to write about the sort of situations which commonly arise in general practice.

I enjoy being in a partnership, and I enjoy the challenge of working things through with my partners in a spirit of mature openness and support with the encouragement of a highly skilled manager. They have encouraged me to develop professionally and have, quite literally, helped to preserve my sanity.

1

Core values and the practice ideals

Key moral and professional stances

These are the issues that give a practice its character, and are expressions of the core beliefs of the practice. We all have core values although we may not think of them as such, and it is these that make us choose to work very hard, or to be laid back, to fight for justice, or to grab for ourselves, to yearn for novelty and truth, or to stick with the familiar. Values such as this may not be easy to identify, but when the general practitioner partnership is faced with choices, or put under stress (i.e. the everyday life of a practice), they will inform how partners think and behave. If your own core values are out of line with the rest of the practice you will feel uncomfortable, and when the chips are down you are likely to want to make different choices from your partners, resulting in principled disagreement. On the other hand, if all of the partners have identical core values you are likely to become a pretty stereotyped and lopsided practice. Some creative tension is good, to keep debate alive and avoid 'groupthink', a state of cosy collusion where no one dares to challenge the party line.

As you work through this book you will be making choices for

Box 1.1: Three of my personal core values

I practise medicine because:

1 _____
  _____

2 _____
  _____

3 _____
  _____

Example 1

Doctor A was approached by a five-doctor partnership to explore the possibility of becoming the sixth partner. They all knew each other very well professionally and Doctor A often did locum work for the partners, with which they were very impressed. They practised medicine in similar ways and all got on well with each other. However, Doctor A had a core value that he should always try to do the best possible job, otherwise he was letting himself down. The other partners felt that having personal boundaries was important, and so set limits on their working. The workaholic Doctor A felt angry that the other partners' 'laziness' would diminish his work (and therefore self-worth) and the partners saw his perfectionism as a threat to their self-defences. Doctor A did not join the partnership.

Example 2

Three doctors of different ages and medical styles, from different cultural and ethnic backgrounds all shared the same core value about the immense worth of individual patients, and a shared sense of spirituality, albeit expressed in three different religious traditions. They formed a very strong partnership.

yourself, which will give you clues to your own core values, but now it may be helpful to spend time reflecting, and write down three key personal core values by which you try to live your professional life (*see* Box 1.1 and Examples 1–3). You may wish to refer to this later.

Example 3

With three children at private school and a big mortgage on his home and surgery building, Doctor B needed money! He was hardworking and independent and greatly valued his family's comfortable lifestyle, which to him was a mark of success. He could not afford to risk a partner not working as hard as he did, so although he had a series of assistants, he never looked for a partner.

The stereotypes and self-labelled identity: the practice culture

The core values of the practice, together with its collective experience and corporate culture, lead to a practice's identity. Obviously, there is a whole spectrum of types and styles of practice but some stereotypes can be identified, and often practices will label themselves as 'friendly' or 'academic', for example. You will see these terms in advertisments, and like those in estate agents, they have double meanings for the cynical (*see* Box 1.2). They may sound like what you want, but are they what they seem?

On a more serious note, many practices have carefully thought through moral, political, or religious stances with which they identify themselves. Consider what type of practice might suit your core values. Do you want to be in a cooperative practice where each person, from cleaner to partner, earns the same and shares decision making? Are all partners paid-up members of the Medical Practitioners' Union taking a solid socialist stand? Does the practice take a particular moral stand, for example, on termination of pregnancy? Would you describe yourself as a 'Christian practice', or for that matter a 'Jewish practice' or is this something you would be looking for? I have not seen 'Muslim practice' or any other religious description attached to a practice yet, although I have known practices informally describing themselves with an ethnic label! Where does legitimate unique identity end and cliquish 'groupthink' begin?

Box 1.2: Types of practice

- 'high earning' also known as money-grubbing
- 'prioritising patient care' also known as working like mad for low profits, with no boundaries
- 'academic' also known as a bit snooty and buggering off to the department of general practice whenever it suits, leaving someone else to do the work
- 'innovative' also known as trying every new fad and project and being restlessly unhappy with everything
- 'involvement with a Primary Care Group' a bunch of politicians who work too hard but are never in the practice, who no one trusts, but earning huge amounts from wheeling and dealing
- 'good humoured' also known as collusive and avoiding conflict and challenge
- 'average friendly' also known as faceless and spineless

Groupthink is a state that any close-knit group of people can get into where their desire to stick together and not rock the boat, overrides their motivation to think clearly and objectively. The group is seen as invulnerable and never wrong, and outsiders are seen with a degree of suspicion. It will be hard to express a view that goes against the 'party line' and so there is an illusion of unanimity. Unfortunately, this leads to a lack of debate and a reluctance to seek outside advice. If a practice ends up like this it can be painful to break out, but the danger of groupthink is that it leads to significant underperformance and therefore poorer patient care.

In many practices, the ethos is not labelled as such, being more an unspoken framework of norms within which members operate, without ever being put into words. The practice may be friendly, caring and hard-working; or disorganised stressed, paranoid and grumpy; respecting the rights of professionals and patients; or self-centred with everyone for themselves. There is also an important balance to be struck between, on the one hand, conflicting values leading to unhelpful confrontation and even open warfare, and on the other, cliquish collusion which, ostrich-like, ignores challenges and rational debate. You can only discover this by talking to people, spending time in the practice and keeping your antennae out.

In the end, all practices are a mixture of good and bad elements, like you, so if you ever find the perfect practice do not join, because you will spoil it!

Training practice status

This is worth considering as an issue in itself, but then as a course organiser I am biased.

Being a training practice carries some professional status and guarantees certain standards, because of the need to be visited for approval every three years. Doctors tend to think of training practices as 'good', but patients tend to prefer non-training practices because of better continuity of care.

In practical terms, keeping to the approved standards for training practices can be very expensive in terms of library and consulting room facilities, for example, and is certainly hard work. There is also a lot of educational work to do, with the trainer having a nominal two sessions (two half days) devoted to teaching as well as attending workshops. On the positive side, the practice gains tremendous enrichment from teaching and the whole team is stimulated to develop as fresh ideas are brought in. Education is very infectious. Although always supernumerary to the service needs of a practice a highly skilled professional such as a general practice registrar (GPR) is a very useful person to have around.

Primary Care Group (PCG) involvement

PCGs vary in their structure and workload, from the level 1 advisory role to the health authority through to the very complex level 3 and, in the future, level 4 primary care trust. They also vary greatly in size. One aspect of this is already all too clear. PCGs generate a tremendous amount of work, with internal corporate issues, commissioning, primary care development and clinical governance. This in turn has its impact on practice workload. This will affect all practices, but there will be varying degrees of impact depending on how actively involved with the workings of the PCG the practice wishes to be. If a practice is very involved, with a partner and practice nurse on the PCG board, for example, this will mean a lot of time away from practice business (this appears to be not well reimbursed). On the other hand, the practice will have more influence at PCG level. Conversely, a practice that wants to stay very clinically focused and not play the political game may not have to be distracted too much by the PCG, but could quickly find itself marginalised. Most practices will fall between these extremes and there are plenty of opportunities to be involved in PCG work. However, if partners disagree about how much time should be spent, PCG involvement could become an obvious source of conflict. This is one issue where discussion is necessary in order to avoid any misunderstanding.

2

The partnership dynamic

Team roles

How many partners there are in a practice and how they work together is obviously basic to how the practice runs, but before you make a rapid decision about a practice, consider both your own and your partners' preferred way of working. Think about how you functioned in the different teams you have experienced.

- Are you good in a team, and why?
- What are your strengths and weaknesses?
- Are you a solitary worker, or a collaborator?
- Are you something of an independent freethinker (others may say a loose cannon)?
- Do you like to have clear rules laid down and work to guidelines and protocols?
- Which role do you tend to play in a team: chair, plant, monitor/ evaluator, team-player (*see* Box 2.1)?

Obviously, it is desirable to have an eclectic mix within the team – it is chaos if everyone is an independent freethinker, but fossilised if no one ever challenges the status quo!

Some practices do psychological profiling of prospective new partners to see if they are likely to fit into their team often by using questionnaires, but most are not quite that organised (or obsessional).

Work by Belbin* on management teams in industry has shown that the best functioning management teams have a chair and a plant and a mix of others (*see* Box 2.1). So it seems that it is good to have someone who has the courage and insight to stir things up a bit and someone else with the calm strength to hold it all together and bring things to a negotiated conclusion. All the different roles are useful in different ways.

Box 2.1: Belbin's group roles

Consider which of the following best describes you in the workplace.

Company worker	conservative, dutiful, predictable
Chair	calm, self-confident, controlled
Shaper	highly strung, outgoing, dynamic
Plant	individualistic, serious-minded, unorthodox
Resource investigator	extrovert, enthusiastic, curious communicative
Monitor/evaluator	sober, unemotional, prudent
Team player	socially orientated, mild, sensitive
Completer/finisher	painstaking, orderly, conscientious, anxious

These terms refer to how people tend to function within a team, and are not personality types, although they may be related to personality. A person with an obsessional personality might function in a particular team as a monitor/evaluator, or as a completer/finisher, or as a company worker, or as a chair, depending on which other roles were being played, so it is possible to adapt to the needs of a team. However, each person will be most comfortable with a particular role, so a team of natural plants is not likely to work.

Belbin RM (1991) *Management Teams: why they succeed or fail.* Butterworth-Heinemann, Oxford.

Number of partners

Obviously, this is key to how a practice works, but for equally obvious practical reasons there is limited room for manoeuvre on this. You will wish to examine these issues when considering prospective practices.

The larger practice

In an inner city area like Newham, a large practice might have four to six partners, although in national terms this should be considered to be medium-sized. There are a number of advantages of a large practice (this is my bias coming out again – ours is a four-partner practice). Sharing of skills and resources within a team allows a wide range of services to be provided and responsibility for running the practice can be shared. There is therefore more scope for teamwork, sharing of stress and efficiency. A larger practice will tend to have more influence at PCG and health authority level than an individual small practice and may therefore be in a stronger position to fight for resources or set local priorities, unless a small practice makes this sort of work a major practice activity.

On the other hand, the larger the number of partners the greater the potential for disagreement with partners over core values, money, or clinical work. To overcome this there will need to be an investment of time to make partnership relationships work and more formal boundaries set to guide how partners interact. As a result, meetings may have to be more formal and management structures more clearly defined, making large practices seem less personal, at least at first.

There is a national trend, although not yet seen in the inner cities, towards the 'superpractice' of 12 or more (occasionally many more) partners in the same practice. As we work more closely together in PCGs and cooperatives this trend may grow, turning the practice from being a small or medium-sized business into a sizeable corporation (*see* Chapter 5). My own view on this was summarised once by a friend of mine who, as a patient, had moved to a town where there were only two practices, each with 12 doctors. She commented, like someone feeling the passing of their youth, 'You can't have your own doctor any more'.

Small practices linked

Some smaller practices prefer to work in a linked but arms'-length relationship. They may share premises, cover each other for on-call work, or share resources or practice staff. At the same time, they remain separate practices with their own financial and management processes. This is very likely to be a way forward for inner city areas where small practices are increasingly working together. Obviously, it is up to each practice to decide in which areas they wish to collaborate and in which they wish to remain separate, and the terms on which they will work (*see* Example 4).

The main advantage of this approach is that you can remain 'just good friends' rather than being 'married', so there is more freedom and flexibility. This may be particularly appropriate for some local circumstances (e.g. where premises pose limitations, or rural geography limits the closeness with which doctors can sensibly work).

There are some drawbacks, however. There will be significant duplication of resources, particularly administratively (e.g. do you each employ a practice manager or club together to share perhaps a more skilled manager?). There will also be less support within each practice and a narrower range of services will be available than in one larger practice (*see* Example 5).

If practices choose to work in this way it is worth asking why.

- Why do they want to work together at all?
- What can't they do on their own?
- Why haven't they formed a full partnership?

It might be that a group of people who really do not get on well have been thrown together by circumstances but feel unable to form a partnership relationship. Perhaps linking smaller practices is a pragmatic halfway house that is without a firm foundation and therefore inherently unstable.

Example 4

By a quirk of history, two practices with two partners each developed a close professional relationship. Each practice had a spare room in their premises. One converted their spare room into a treatment room, whereas the other converted theirs into a counselling room. By an arrangement of sharing premises and jointly employing a sessional counsellor they were then both able to offer minor surgery and counselling services to their patients. It is easy to see this arrangement developing closer links between the practices, in a European Union style of 'ever closer union'.

Example 5

In the 'Golden Age' of general practice before the 1990 imposed contract (why do we lock ourselves into this negative thinking – the 'Golden Age' does not always have to be in the past – and why do so many of us still mutter about the political debates of a decade ago?) there was a Red Book payment called the 'group practice allowance', to encourage single-handed doctors to work more closely together. So it was that four doctors working independently in the same health centre decided to form loose links. They decided to share a practice manager and administrative staff, but remain independent doctors. This worked for a while but because the doctors continued to work and think as individuals it became very hard for them to agree, and they soon spent most of the time arguing. They had not put enough investment into joint working. They returned to being single-handed practices after the rather weak glue of the group practice allowance was abolished.

Small practices

Although single-handed practice is not really the major concern of this book, it is worth mentioning that it has its own attractions as a flexible and independent way of working, and will remain a significant feature of the general practice picture, particularly in inner city areas, but two- and to some extent three-handed practices have their own unique partnership issues. With nowhere to hide and no one to mediate, the practice hinges critically on the nature of the relationship between the partners. If they can work openly and honestly together then all will go well, but if there is significant disagreement then 'divorce' is all too common. For example, within Newham, an area with a high proportion of single-handed practices, many of these have arisen out of partnership disputes within two- and three-handed practices. On the other hand, there are examples where a small partnership is robust.

Dynamics between partners

The way partners relate to each other in both formal and informal settings (e.g. in partners' meetings and over lunch) is vital to consider, but may be very hard to pin down or assess with clarity. The key question is can this group of individuals, including you, find a way to work together comfortably and respect each other?

Issues like joining a husband and wife who are partners, or partnerships with open conflict between partners, are situations which one would have to be very careful with, although both can actually work well. Talk to partners and ex-partners and anyone else who may be well-informed, to discover as much as possible about internal politics and personalities. In the end gut feeling may be the best guide (*see* Example 6).

It may be worthwhile asking partners how they deal with conflict or strong feelings within the team. This would reveal the partnership that tends to avoid conflict, and will also indicate if partners have considered the issue of difficult discussions and the feelings that arise. If there is a culture of open discussion and acknowledgement of each other's feelings and opinions the under-lying dynamic between the partners is likely to be secure and confident (*see* Example 7).

Some more formal models of how the practice runs and partner-ship dynamics can be pinned down fairly easily and give clues to the less formal aspects. I have outlined some of these in the following sections.

Example 6
Doctor C joined a practice with three other doctors, D, E and F. Unknown to her, D and E were finding it hard to get on with F, who had joined the practice only 10 months earlier. C ignored her gut feelings of unease but soon after joining it became clear that she was also having problems relating to F and was tending to side with D and E. Eventually, after much heartache on both sides F, who was struggling with marriage problems which he had tried to hide from the practice, moved on to another practice and C, D and E continued as a partnership. All those involved were haunted by these problems for several years.

Example 7
Doctor G was invited to become a partner in the practice in which she had been a registrar. The four existing partners were robust with each other and partners' meetings tended to end in votes with a predictable two and two split. In effect, there were two opposing parties within the partnership. Doctor G was well aware of this when she agreed to join. She had a non-confrontational but strong character and enjoyed having the balance of power. She quickly took the role of chair and the whole partnership dynamic softened.

The senior partner as executive

In this relatively simple model, one partner, perhaps the 'senior' partner, leads on most decisions and chairs the partnership. He works quite closely with the practice manager, if there is one, and will delegate tasks to partners as necessary. This sounds autocratic but may work well with a sensitive executive who is a natural lead figure and has appropriate management skills. Obviously, the other partners need to feel comfortable with a more subordinate role, but are freer to indulge other medical interests (*see* Figure 2.1).

A key advantage of this model is that lines of decision making are clear within the practice which helps the practice manager, and

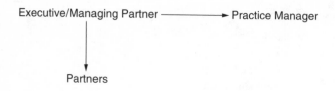

Figure 2.1 The senior partner model.

it will be clear to those outside the practice, such as the health authority, who to relate to. However, this can put a lot of pressure on the executive partner, who may well need a lower clinical load and extra time to do the management work.

On the negative side, having one powerful figure within the partnership can lead to tension and resentment. At some point, a young lion–old lion conflict is very likely, but then no single dynamic will last for ever. Practices evolve. However, this model limits the management skill and time of the practice to those of the executive, so that other partners may have no opportunity (or are not forced by circumstances) to develop these skills. What then happens when the executive is on holiday, or ill with his ulcer, or is convicted of fraud?

Democracy and shared responsibility

In this model, the partners all work together and have equal power within the partnership, but divide the responsibility for the key management functions between them. Each partner will make simple decisions in his/her own area of responsibility in conjunction with the practice manager, but for larger issues they will bring the matter to the partners' meeting for a full discussion. This is a type of 'Cabinet' structure (*see* Figure 2.2).

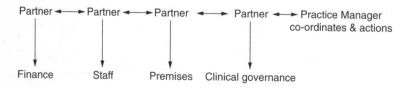

Figure 2.2 The shared responsibility model.

The advantages of this system are that it is fair to each partner and it respects each person's strengths. It is possible to match the tasks to a partner's skills, for example, making the monitor/ evaluator responsible for clinical governance, or the obsessive with financial skill in charge of finance. The management load is spread between all the partners and all are involved in some leadership, building trust within the practice, and capitalising on the breadth of skills available. Rapid response to change becomes possible with partners working autonomously in their own areas of responsibility with the practice manager.

There is no such thing as a free lunch. The downside of a shared responsibility system is that a large management team can lead to confusion. It may be difficult to deal with issues that cross boundaries of partners' responsibility, and there must be a high degree of trust between partners. To maintain this there will need to be a lot of discussion time, and a self-confident manager. Another disadvantage is that not all partners may wish to be heavily involved in running the practice.

Management team within a partnership.

This is similar to the model described in the previous section, but with some partners choosing to stay out of managing the practice. This will be very flexible to partners' needs, but the back seat partners may feel marginalised and disempowered. Meanwhile, the managing partners may feel resentful about their extra work and responsibility (*see* Figure 2.3).

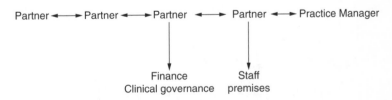

Figure 2.3 The management team model.

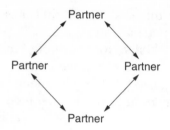

Figure 2.4 The total democratic model.

Everyone makes decisions together

As Figure 2.4 suggests, this can be a pleasant, friendly way of doing things. On the surface, it sounds attractive. Everyone is consulted, and then you either act on the consensus of all the partners, or the will of the majority, depending on how you want to work it. This may be feasible for a very small practice, but in a medium- or large-sized practice it would take a long time to make decisions if all the partners had to agree on everything, unless you are going to spend a lot of time in partners' meetings. If a large practice, or even a medium-sized practice, adopts this type of decision making it may suggest problems in the partnership dynamic. Perhaps the partners have not really thought through management issues, and run the practice as a cottage industry rather than a modern business. Perhaps they lack trust in each other, or are unhappy about the risk of making independent decisions without discussion with others. Of course, you may feel that these so-called problems are in fact excellent qualities for doctors, and could be termed sensitivity to others, a respect for human scale values, and focusing on people rather than processes. It depends on your viewpoint.

There are no right or wrong ways of doing things, only different choices.

Joint responsibility for decisions

Being in partnership means you share legal responsibilities. For example, you jointly employ staff and are therefore jointly responsible for employment law issues. You are also jointly liable for most practice debts. (Interestingly, you are now not jointly liable for tax debts, only for your own share of the partnership tax.) So, if one partner unfairly dismisses a staff member, the whole partnership can be taken to an industrial tribunal, or if one partner runs up a huge bill on the practice account, the partnership will still have to pay. Thus the critical question is do you trust your partners? Will you be happy to accept majority voting and majority decisions, even when you disagree?

How will formal decisions be made?

Whichever management model you adopt you will still need to agree on a mechanism by which formal partnership decisions are made. One possibility is working by consensus, where all the partners agree informally before decisions are made, or you may prefer to formalise it with voting and implement actions by unanimous vote only.

This system would rapidly become unworkable in all but the smallest practices (try getting any group of general practitioners to all agree on anything!) and thus, as with the ever-expanding European Union, there will have to be some decision making by majority vote. (You might want to be a bit careful in a three-partner practice where two partners are married!) If you use a voting system, you will still need to work out which decisions will be decided by majority vote, and which by unanimous vote. Major policy issues, such as a change in practice area, would probably need to be unanimous, and any change in the partnership deed, the partners' governing contract with each other, has to be unanimous. Less important issues could be made on a majority basis, but it can be hard to draw the line between major and minor decisions. Perhaps the partnership deed should include some relevant examples.

You might even want to consider a system of qualified majority voting where, for example, a two to three majority is needed – this can become very complicated. Perhaps it would be wise to take some time to reflect on what each of these systems says about the dynamics of the partnership? (*See* Examples 8 and 9.)

Example 8

A five-doctor practice used to work with an executive partner system and their partnership shares were weighted so that the executive partner drew a slightly larger share than the others. As the work of a modern practice grew, the partners changed the way they worked to a shared responsibility system. Before long, the four previously junior partners realised that the existing partnership shares were unjust with shared responsibility, but knew that to change shares would require unanimous agreement, which would not be easy to get! However, money was in limited supply for two of them, and they felt that to keep the current shares could represent an illegal sale of goodwill (see p. 35). At a tense and frank partnership meeting they confronted the issue and with a unanimous decision they amended the shares to reflect true workload.

Example 9

In a three-partner practice, one partner was on long-term sick leave. On her return, she found that the other two partners had made a decision to spend £2000 on a new autoclave, which she felt was not really needed. This was not, however, a major policy decision, and their partnership deed provided for simple majority voting for routine decisions, so she 'bit the bullet' and paid her share.

Practice manager or practice administrator?

The person in charge of managing the practice organisation is pivotal, and influences both the work of the partners and the style and culture of the practice. No two practice managers seem to do quite the same job, and there are, in fact, two reasonably distinct species in this genus that are fairly easy to identify. Confusingly, both are called **practice manager**. You may be happier with one or other type depending on how you wish to work, but if you employ the wrong one for your practice, the effects could become very uncomfortable. (But *see* Box 2.2.)

The first type could be called a *true manager*. These individuals will be proactive in making decisions and have a professional

---

Box 2.2: NJVRS: the need to be responsible

I'm a doctor and don't want to be burdened with administration, and lack management skills	It's my practice so I should be fully involved in ensuring it works. I can learn the skills

NJVRS, non-judgemental rating scales (see Introduction).

---

management approach, managing the practice and its various components (finance, staff, premises and equipment, time, systems, teams, etc.) rather than being managed by the partners; in addition taking a strong strategic role in the practice. They will obviously have strong management skills and training, and will have sound assertiveness skills. They are expensive to employ, but are very good at encouraging innovation and change and, through this, practice and team development. A *true manager* will take a lot of the administrative burdens from the partners and may well be able to increase income; for example, by perfecting internal systems, such as the item of service claiming routine. Also, you may find that maternity or contraceptive fee claims are increased, or the manager may well know ways of using the Red Book to your advantage. The details of the Red Book are esoteric and most doctors do not fully understand it (or have the time or motivation to learn about it), especially items like advance leave payments, dispensing regulations or the fee for arrest of a dental haemorrhage. A good *true manager* will navigate the Red Book with some skill. This would, of course, help to offset the high salary. (*See* Example 10.)

The second type of practice manager could be called a *practice administrator*. This professional will run the administrative side of the practice and do (or delegate) the routine tasks, such as the payroll and keeping informed on income and expenditure, and Red Book payments. However, unlike the *true manager*, the *practice administrator* would not be expected to take a strategic view of practice development or seek to 'manage' the partners. Rather, the partners would very much remain in control of the business, and not encourage the *administrator* to make proactive innovation. Although often very experienced, *administrators* are generally paid

> **Example 10**
>
> A five-partner practice was struggling to keep up with its management work. They were an innovative training practice with a manager approaching retirement who worked as an *administrator*. When he retired, a new manager, very much of the *true manager* type was appointed. She was able to rebuild the organisation and help progress practice development, and make a significant difference to the partners' stress levels.

on a lower salary scale, and are more likely to be affordable by smaller practices. They are also less threatening to general practitioners who feel that the partners own the business and should therefore run it.

If you want to be very much in control then an *administrator* may be right for you, particularly if you have strong management skills and time to spend on these. On the other hand, if you want to have an innovative practice but feel you lack management skills and experience you may prefer a *true manager*. (*See* Example 11.)

> **Example 11**
>
> A well-established practice with one principal and two assistants felt a need to innovate. They needed new premises and wanted to expand their team and the services they offered. They appointed a new and enthusiastic manager who had a lot of experience as a deputy practice manager in a practice in another village, and wanted to further his career. After a few months it became clear that the principal had difficulty handing over control, making staff decisions without talking to the manager, and not including him in discussions with the health authority about the new building. The manager felt he had less responsibility than in his previous job and so moved on to another job.

Attitudes to part-time or job-share

Many of us like the idea of job-share or part-time working, with its flexibility to fit around family, academic or other commitments and the potential for lower stress levels. It seems likely that this type of employment will become more common in the future despite the lower earning potential, but this will have an impact on practices.

More partners means more relationships within the partnership. This makes working relationships harder to negotiate, with more potential for disagreement, and greater need for more formal frameworks within the practice. You might need to have a more formal committee structure for partnership meetings, or more structured approaches to communication. However, having more people in the team increases the skills base, so you may be able to broaden your practice services. Part-timers often say they have less influence within the practice, and full-timers often perceive part-timers as having less commitment and of not being able to take the pace.

Assistantships

Assistants are not principals, and so are not on the local medical list, but they are doctors who have completed general practitioner training and have a Joint Committee on Postgraduate Training in General Practice (JCPTGP) certificate. They are employed by the practice, and sadly the history of assistants is littered with stories of

Example 12

Doctor K had been working in general practice for 20 years as an assistant. She had appreciated the lower level of responsibility as she had spent time bringing up her family. The job was also more secure than locum work. However as the only woman in a practice of four male doctors she ended up being asked to run family planning and child surveillance services, and did most of the gynaecology work. When her family grew up she wanted more varied work and more responsibility, as now she had more experience than most of the partners. Other practices seemed unwilling to offer her a partnership because of her age and relatively narrow skills. She felt trapped and exploited in a role she had long outgrown, and the partners kept on offloading her with work they did not want to do.

exploitation of doctors by doctors, with low pay, high workloads and little job security (*see* Example 12). There are, of course, examples where the arrangement works well (*see* Example 13).

- Would you work as an assistant, with little control over your work and relatively low pay, but flexibility (e.g. to change jobs) and limited commitment?
- Would you want to employ such a person? As the employing partnership you would get some reimbursement for the salary from the health authority in the form of an assistant allowance.

Example 13

Doctor J was unattached and enjoyed an active outdoor life. Soon after qualifying he had spent time in Canada climbing and canoeing and doing hospital locum work. He moved back to Snowdonia, Wales and completed general practitioner training. He then continued to pursue his climbing career, funding it through a part-time assistant job in a local practice. This also enabled him to go on interesting expeditions as the team doctor.

'Salaried partners'

There is no such organism as a 'salaried partner'. A partner is a self-employed individual who owns a share of the business and draws a share of the profits, usually a percentage share, the exact value of which will vary with the profits. Someone drawing a fixed salary is an employee, with different tax liabilities and employment rights. A salaried person has rights to go to an industrial tribunal and sick leave rights, for example. They also are subject to the terms of a contract, for example to work certain set hours. A partner could, however, draw a fixed share (a fixed sum rather than a percentage) of the profit. He is then legally a partner, with the full rights of a partner (e.g. to see the accounts), and is a principal in general practice, but without some of the financial risks and benefits of being an ordinary percentage share partner. Having a fixed share might be an alternative to a percentage share in the period leading up to parity because it would provide a clearly defined income without having to calculate the vagaries of income streams and expenses.

If you receive a salary rather than a fixed share of profits you are an employee, with different rights, but with no authority to have any say in the running of the business. The term 'salaried partner' has been used in the past to appoint an employee doctor but still claim basic practice allowance. This is exploitation.

In the future it is likely that trusts and primary care groups will create more salaried posts, which might be attractive to new general practitioners. At present, there are only a few examples of these 'salaried option' jobs. I would suggest to anyone considering such a post to consider:

- the length of contract and job security
- the employer and how they might treat you
- different tax rules for employed people compared to the self-employed
- the risk that you might undersell yourself with a relatively low salary.

Of course I am a partner in a practice that suits me well so I am bound to be wary of anything new, but which may well be right for you.

Patients and personal lists

How will you allocate the patients? Personal lists, where patients are restricted as far as possible to seeing their registered doctor, encourage continuity of care but are administratively difficult (*see* Box 2.3). What do you do in an emergency when the patient's doctor is away, for example? It may be worthwhile overcoming these problems if the partners work in very different ways, but it will be harder to develop and audit practice policy and protocols with doctors working quite separately. Do you want to deny patients the right to choose to see a different doctor for a particular problem? Personal lists also make it difficult to develop areas of clinical interest within the practice. Minor surgery, for example, has to be done by a partner who is on the minor surgery list. Will a minor surgery

---

Box 2.3: NJVRS: the need to be the patient's source of help

My patients should obtain personal care from me because I know them and their families

We all follow the same protocols, so it should be any port in a storm for the patient

---

partner carry out procedures on other partners' lists? If not, for the sake of personal lists, you will reduce services and restrict income. If so, the logic of personal lists starts to break down. There are many similar situations that make a rigid personal list system hard to maintain.

Mutual assessment periods and progression to parity

All parties will be keen to establish firm secure working relationships as quickly as possible when a partner joins a practice, but will also be wary of making a firm commitment too soon. Sometimes partnerships, like relationships do not always work out. It is therefore wise to look at agreeing a mutual assessment period at the end of which either side can walk away from the deal without rancour or blame. This gives both sides a pressure-free period to see how things go, but how long should this be? Clearly, this must be agreed. Like engagements, if the mutual assessment period is too short you risk making a big mistake (partnership splits are as traumatic as divorce, but more expensive), but if too long, it sends a message of reluctance to make a commitment, and a fear that the new person will be rejected. He or she will be a full legal partner during this time, on whatever share is agreed, but may have less power in the partnership.

Mutual assessment is not the same as progression to parity, which is the length of time it will take for the new partner to draw a share equal to everyone else, after prior shares (*see* p.31) and pro rata rates for part-timers. The progression to parity could start at the same time as a mutual assessment period or after the final commitment is made. The justification for progression to parity is that a new partner will not take as much responsibility for running the practice as the existing partners. Exactly what share a new partner draws during the period to parity is a matter of negotiation, but no partner should draw less than a third of the drawings of the highest earner (pro rata for part-timers). Some practices are happy to do away with progression to parity altogether, and at the other extreme, periods longer than three years are suspect.

Restrictive covenants on leaving

A restricted covenant clause is a section of a partnership deed that restricts what a partner who leaves can do after leaving. You might, for example, agree that a partner who leaves may not treat patients who are on the practice list at the time they leave for at least one year. This type of covenant may safeguard the practice if a partner leaves with his list of 2000 patients and sets up shop next door, but may be unfair to a new person who might want to leave if the situation becomes unsatisfactory but still wants to work locally. If the covenant is too broad, for example you would not be permitted to see any patients living within five miles of the practice for five years in an urban area, then the whole covenant is void and unenforceable. In summary, restrictive covenants must be fair and reasonable to both sides.

Compulsory expulsion

In the partnership deed, there will be a clause you should include about the circumstances in which you might be required to resign from the practice. These are worth considering. Many of the causes are obvious (e.g. if you are struck off the medical register), but there may be conditions where you might feel expulsion would be inappropriate or discriminatory (see Example 14). You may never imagine that these clauses might be used, but it is worthwhile contemplating about what might lead to expulsion.

What is a 'hanging' offence? Ensure there is a clause to cover the partnership if one partner does commit 'treason against the partnership' (*see* Example 15), but also ensure that partners are not inadvertently exposed to unfair expulsion.

There is, of course, no recourse to an industrial tribunal for unfair dismissal. You are self-employed.

Example 14

In a practice of four doctors, one partner, Doctor L, became unexpectedly ill with an acute severe depression. He had no past history but was admitted to hospital as an informal patient, although the severity of the illness would have warranted compulsory admission if he had refused to go. After a year, Doctor L was able to return to work full-time. However, the partnership deed indicated that if a partner was compulsorily admitted under sections 2 or 3 of the Mental Health Act 1983 he could be expelled from the partnership. There were other reasonable provisions for sick-leave for physical or mental illness. At the time the deed was drawn up no one really looked at this clause – it would never happen to them. When Doctor L recovered it was felt that the clause discriminated against mental illness, and was removed, much to the relief of Doctor L who continues to live with the knowledge that his depression could recur.

Example 15

In a six-partner urban practice five partners got on well, but one partner, Doctor K, was isolated. He disagreed with the others on many partnership issues, and staff found him hard to deal with. His presence seemed to paralyse the practice, but because he had not breached any part of the partnership deed he could not be required to leave.

3

Owning or leasing the premises

This is an extremely complex issue, which can only really be touched on here, but is probably less important for new partners than one might think – which is surprising given the amount of money involved.

Own (and control) the premises

If the partners own the premises they will have control and responsibility for them.

In order to own a share of the property, a partner would have to raise the capital, which could easily amount to anything up to £300 000 at 1999 prices. This is likely to be a loan with interest payments, and when you compare this to house mortgage costs it appears witheringly expensive. However, the interest payments should be covered by the cost rent or notional rent payments from the health authority to the practice for the privilege of using your privately owned building for NHS work, in seeing NHS patients. Interestingly, if you do too much private work in your building (in excess of 10% of practice income) the health authority will reduce their payments. With the interest thus taken care of you only have to worry about the capital invested. You might choose to pay this off gradually so that when you retire you can sell your share of the building to the next partner, thus providing you with an agreeable little lump sum. Alternatively, if this type of investment is not for you, you could maintain the loan as a business debt, in which case you do not have to sink money into the property but you will not get anything back on retirement, and you continue to have a massive debt until you have got someone to buy it from you. Banks may be reluctant to allow the second option.

When a partner leaves, his/her share can be bought by the other partners or by his/her successor at the current market rate, and they will then be responsible for rent payments. The leaving partner, on selling, will get back his/her original investment plus any growth due to property price inflation. You may also wish to put a clause in the partnership deed to say that the leaving partner does not have to sell his/her share for less than they paid for it, in order to avoid negative equity problems in the event of a property slump.

Thus, taking out a loan for £300 000 could be viewed as a pension investment which could be quite worthwhile, like getting the interest payments on your mortgage paid by the health authority, while you stand to gain, effectively free of cost, any growth in the capital investment, with a guarantee that you will not lose.

However, with owning the practice property comes the responsibility for it, and the risk associated with a huge investment. Having such a large financial commitment may restrict a partner, particularly at the start of his/her career as a principal, when he/she may feel they might wish to move practices at some point. New partners may also be justifiably nervous of the risk, given the pace of change in the NHS.

In some practices, some partners own the building with their associates taking no role in it, depending on their personal feelings about financial risk. (*See* Example 16.)

Example 16

A five-doctor practice worked from a newly built inner city surgery that cost £1.2 million to build. Originally, four partners had raised

continued

capital of £300 000 each to buy the property. The fifth partner had decided to stay out of the deal because she was near to retirement anyway. After she retired, a new partner joined whose spouse worked for the Foreign Office. He was likely to reach full ambassador status in the next few years, so the new partner could well move on from the practice, and therefore did not wish to buy into the premises.

A few years later one of the partners resigned. He owned part of the building and tried to sell this to his replacement. However, the replacement partner again had good reasons not to buy in. The other partners did not want to have the resigning partner continuing to own a share of the premises, and he did not want to have anything more to do with the practice either. The situation was resolved by the three existing owners extending their capital investment by a further £100 000 each to buy out the resigning partner. Thus out of five partners, three have a £400 000 share in the building, whereas two partners feel they have the flexibility they need.

Lease

Leased premises are less of a financial risk, as the cost of the lease will normally be covered by payments from the health authority under the rent and rates scheme (covered in section 51, the most complex of all Red Book sections). Thus, each quarter, the landlord is paid the rent on the lease by the practice and the health authority reimburses the practice with a rent payment. Usually, but not invariably, the payments will net out, so that the practice neither loses nor gains. However, with lower risk there will be less control over the building and you become subject to the terms of the lease. For example, you might have to completely redecorate every year at the practice's expense.

As the lease is a shared responsibility of the partnership as a whole, and not of individual partners as individual capital investments would be, there is no feeling of individuals being tied down but only the landlord ever makes any money out of the arrangement. (*See* Example 17.)

Example 17

A four-doctor practice moved into a new building worth £900 000. The property was owned by a developer who had financed the project and worked on the design with the partners. Rent was agreed at £90 000 per year which was paid by the practice to the developer, and from the health authority to the practice. Routine maintenance will be dealt with by the practice, and paid for out of a rent supplement which the health authority pays to the practice, so the practice retains some control over the building. There remains some uncertainty about what will happen at the rent review in three years when the developer can increase the rent on the advice of an independent surveyor, but the health authority will have to impose whatever the then district valuer assesses the rent to be. There may be difficult negotiations.

However, the practice has got the building it wanted without being tied down to the risk and commitment of a £900 000 loan.

Rent

Some practices work in community trust property, and pay rent which is reimbursed by the health authority in the same way as described above. Thus, there is little or no financial risk to the practice, unless the trust goes bankrupt, and no net cost either. There is therefore room for flexibility for partners to join and leave the practice. Links with primary healthcare team members are likely to be good. However, the practice will have no control over the building and how it is serviced. They may have to use trust staff, in a shared switchboard for example, and will be subject to trust managers' decisions about the building (*see* Example 18). You may also have to pay a service charge which is not reimbursed by the health authority.

Example 18

A three doctor practice working in a trust health centre wanted to put up some shelving in the practice library. They were faced with a delay of five months while the trust decided whether it could agree to this request, as it constituted an alteration to the building!

4

Financial issues

In this chapter I consider issues related to how National Health Service income is allocated and managed. (Note that the Appendix lists all the main sources of NHS income in general practice.)

Pooling income

A basic decision is what income will be allocated in partnership shares and what will be allocated in other ways. Most of the income will be pooled. That is, it is put into a central pot where it is set against expenses and profit calculated, which is then distributed in profit-sharing ratios. Some income, however, may not be apportioned in this way and is termed a *prior share*, because it is shared out, in proportions not related to partnership shares, prior to the calculation of profit. For example, if two out of four partners own the building, then the health authority rent income would almost certainly be given as a prior share to the owning partners, in proportion to their share of ownership of the building. This income would offset their mortgage costs. This is just as the non-owning partners have no financial interest in the building or claim on the rent. However, if the partnership as a whole owned a lease on the building, the rent would go into the pool, and be offset against the cost of the lease which would be paid out of the practice pool. These examples are straightforward, but some income streams could reasonably be pooled or kept as prior shares depending on your point of view. Thus, earnings from a partner's outside post as a clinical assistant could be kept as a prior share, because that partner does the work. Or, it could be shared in the pool because during the time the partner is being a clinical assistant, the other partners have to do his practice work on his behalf. There are no firm rules, only what you negotiate.

Which aspects of the practice income will be pooled, and therefore shared out in profit-sharing ratios, and which will be retained individually by partners? Seniority payments are often taken as prior shares, although younger partners may not see why older colleagues should not pool this income. Postgraduate Education Allowance (PGEA) may be pooled, but would it be fair if a lazy partner who never did any education should bring down everyone's income? Should the minor surgery partner keep all the income from that source, or should this be shared out?

Consider the list of income sources (*see* Appendix) and decide which of these you are going to share in profit-sharing ratios (e.g. capitation and targets are commonly pooled), and which you will retain individually (e.g. PGEA is often taken as a prior share). Some practices pool all income, some allocate in very complex ways in order to meet individual circumstances.

Attitudes to outside work

A particular problem is what are you going to do with income from outside appointments, such as:

- clinical assistantships
- course organiser appointments
- insurance reports
- police work
- nursing home retainers.

If you pool income, will you redistribute the practice work accordingly so that income reflects workload? It would be unfair to pool a partner's nursing home retainer but insist that she continues to do the same amount of work within the practice. Another problem arises when time spent on an outside job earns less than could be earned from surgery work. A fee for running an education workshop would be far lower than the income generated if the time were spent carrying out liquid nitrogen minor surgery, for example. (*See* Example 19.)

Indeed, do you want outside appointments? Some practices do not allow it. Outside appointments can generate a lot of income but cause considerable disruption to surgery work and patient care. Being a police surgeon is said (perhaps by those who do not know) to be a licence to print money. However, this can mean going out at night or during mid surgery for an indefinite period of time without warning. You might need to have locum cover for this situation which may be more expensive than the money you earn. Some appointments (e.g. course organiser) are relatively poorly paid as well as being time-consuming. Could you tolerate a partner doing this extra work? (*See* Example 20.)

When considering outside appointments, you need to balance workload, income, personal enjoyment, development of skills, and patient care.

Outside work may be done in practice time with reorganisation of the workload, or may be carried out outside practice time. Either way, there are issues about who covers the routine surgery work.

Example 19

In a five-doctor practice, partners' outside appointments include educational and nursing home appointments. Income from these is pooled, but the partners with the outside appointments do one surgery per week fewer than the others to compensate.

Example 20

In a four-doctor practice each partner does seven surgeries a week. Outside appointments include occupational health and hospital practitioner posts. These sessions are done in addition to practice work and so the income is not shared.

Pooling expenses

Just as income may or may not be pooled, so also with expenses to a lesser extent. Main practice expenses (e.g. staff salaries) will usually be paid from the pooled income, but what about more personal items like Medical Defence Union/Medical Protection Society expenses or car expenditure, when individual partners may be able to obtain different deals? You will probably not all want to drive the same type of car, and different cars cost different amounts so why should you share out the expenses equally? What about course fees and professional memberships? The fair answer will depend on how you allocate income such as PGEA. You could argue that the practice will pay GMC (General Medical Council) registration fees as it is a flat rate fee per doctor and you have a mutual interest in ensuring each other's registration is paid.

It is usual to be able to reach reasonable agreement on expenditure issues, but it is easy to see how the partnership deed could become quite detailed (*see* Example 21).

Example 21

A four-doctor practice used a deputising service for night calls. On their nights on-call two of the partners did all their own calls up to midnight and then handed over to the deputising service. Of the other partners, one covered telephone advice only on her evenings on-call, and one switched everything over to the deputising service at 7.00pm. The partners agreed that the deputising expenses should not be pooled and divided in partnership shares, but should be divided up in proportion to the number of calls done by the service on the nights that each partner was on-call. This was an administrative nightmare, not least in keeping track of exactly what use each partner made of the deputising service, however the arrangement did accommodate all the partners' needs.

Partnership shares

How will you allocate pooled profit?

• Equally?

- What about part-timers?
- What about people doing different on-call arrangements?
- Will the executive partner have a larger share, or lighter clinical load?

These are key questions to consider in allocating pooled income. It may at first sight be fairest to divide income equally, but justice requires that share should truly reflect workload.

Sale of goodwill

If you buy a shop, you would pay for the buildings, stock and other assets, but also, quite properly, for goodwill. This is the reputation and customer base of the shop, and can be given a monetary value to reflect its importance to the business. In general practice there is an equivalent – and it is illegal. If a single-handed doctor takes on a partner he might say that because everyone knows him and he set up the practice, he should have a larger share of the profits. In effect, the new partner is buying 'goodwill' from the existing partner. This is a form of exploitation. The Local Medical Committees (LMCs) are always on the look out for this, even in its hidden form where time or workload is used to buy goodwill. A senior partner cannot plan to see half as many patients as his partner and claim the same share of the profit. Profit share must always reflect actual workload as far as possible. You can, of course, be paid more for additional administrative, or clinical work. When a new partner joins, it is assumed that he/she will have initially a lower clinical and administrative workload, in particular. This is the basis for progression to parity but if progression is too slow (e.g. more than three years), it will be interpreted as a sale of goodwill (*see* Example 8: revisited). At all times, it should be clear why people are drawing their particular level of share, and it should be obvious to those outside that it is an attempt to reflect work carried out.

Example 8: revisited

This five-doctor practice used to work with an executive partner system and their partnership shares were weighted so that the executive partner drew a slightly larger share than the others. As the work of the partners changed they swapped to a shared responsibility system. Before long, the four previously junior partners realised that the existing partnership shares were not only unjust but could represent an illegal sale of goodwill. At a tense and frank partnership meeting they confronted the issue and with a unanimous decision they altered the shares to reflect true workload. Having a working knowledge of the legal position certainly helped to focus the discussion.

Showing accounts to the interviewee

At some point, a prospective partner will need to see the accounts in order to make a decision about the practice. Partners will need to balance their desire to appear open and financially sound with an equally reasonable desire to keep information confidential.

Prospective partners should balance their need to see the accounts against an appearance of seeming suspicious or money-grubbing. It may be difficult to balance these competing issues; but a wise practice will show the accounts to any prospective partner who asks, and a wise applicant will not ask to see these immediately and will reassure the partners that he/she will treat the information with respect and confidentiality. Obviously, it is important to look carefully at the figures with a qualified accountant, and this should be mentioned to the partners. (*See* Examples 22 and 23.)

You can learn a lot from accounts about a practice:

- how the partnership works
- how organised they are
- how efficient they are and, of course,
- get an idea of how financially sound they are.

Example 22

Doctor M was hoping to join a four-partner practice and at the second interview asked to see the accounts. He was presented with a brown envelope containing a variety of documentation, including income and expenditure accounts for the previous three months, and a handful of bank statements! Despite this evident chaos he joined the practice, and discovered that the culture of colluding to avoid conflict was widespread. No one had wanted to tackle the financial situation because they did not want to admit that they were in over their heads and did not know where to start. Anyway, they all drew a reasonable income each month so there was no perceived pressing need. After partnership changes, practice manager changes, and a general practitioner contract change, the practice gradually sorted out its finances, through a steady process of education and change management.

Example 23

Doctor N had just finished her registrar year and had been approached to join a local six-partner teaching practice. When she examined the accounts she found substantial profits as a result of high deprivation payments and item of service fees. The accountants were specialist medical accountants who had produced a commentary on the accounts suggesting ways in which efficiency could be improved. The accounts also showed that a full range of services was being offered. Doctor N was sure that at this practice her financial future would be secure, but she also could see from the high list size that she was going to have to work hard.

Banking policy and accounts

The partnership deed will specify the partnership's bankers (who should be local, for convenience), and accountants (who may or may not be local). There is a lot to be said for using accountants with a special interest in general practitioner accounts, given the complexity of the Red Book. Accountants will sort out yearly accounts (or quarterly if required, at a price) and deal with partnership taxation, and offer advice on financial issues if required. Professional fees of accountants vary considerably so it is worth considering inviting estimates from different firms if the bill seems high.

It used to be the case that partners could be held personally liable for any unpaid tax from any partner's share of the profits, but now, under self-assessment, you will only be liable for the tax on your share of the profits. However, each partner can still be held liable for the whole of any other partnership debt if the partnership defaults.

As a partner, you will pay tax twice a year, and your accountant will advise you on how to make provision for this in a practice tax reserve. You can obtain tax relief on a wide variety of personal expenses, which again your accountant will advise you on, but these must be genuine expenses. If any of your partners are inflating their claims, the Inland Revenue can order an investigation of all the partners' expenses, and require inspection of records for the previous seven years. This is usually at great expense in terms of accountants' fees. Make sure, therefore, that all the partners follow practice policy on personal expenses as advised by the accountants.

Check accounts carefully with someone who understands them, but also check the bank details and partnership deed to see if all partners are named on the bank account. Who will be signatories; all partners, or just some? How many partners will be needed to sign a cheque? If everyone must sign everything you will have problems if someone is away, but on the other hand, make sure you do not just have one signatory, or, even worse produce a rubber stamp signature of the only signatory! It has been done and you cannot reclaim the money you lose in fraud!

Private patients

Unless you have an unusual skill, such as laser tattoo removal, the scope for private work in Newham is limited. However, some patients may still see you privately. For example, overseas visitors from countries without a reciprocal agreement with non-emergency health needs are not covered by the NHS, so you may be asked to see them privately. Relatives of registered patients who have come from abroad might fit in this category. Some doctors have moral objections to private work, or at least find it hard to ask ill people for money (*see* Box 4.1), so it is a good idea to have a working policy on how much to charge and how to collect the money.

- How will you distribute money gained from private work?
- Will you keep it individually, or share it in the pool?
- When will you see private patients, during ordinary surgeries or in your own time?

Box 4.1: NJVRS: feelings about private medicine

Care should be on the basis of need, not ability to pay, so private medicine is morally wrong, and I want no part in it

Why shouldn't people with money be able to use it on their health, and why shouldn't I gain from this too?

5

How hard do you want to work?

Workload

How do you feel about hard work? What level of workload is acceptable to you? These are questions that people do not address adequately, and when they do, they do not always give honest answers. You and your partners need to balance patient care with income and your own sanity. This means you need to discuss both issues thoroughly, and reach a reasonable compromise which you can all live with. Too many partnerships break up over the issue of perceived workload.

The balance is set something like this:

- generally, the higher the list size the greater the income
- but the higher the list the greater the workload
- the higher the workload the greater the pressure to restrict patient care.

Your own position on these axes is more important than negotiating particular workloads. The workaholics will always exceed their work time, whatever is agreed (*see* Example 1: revisited), and the bone idle will always tend to dodge their

Example 1: revisited
When Doctor A decided not to join the five-doctor practice (see Example 1), it was clear that his perfectionism set him a high workload, which he could tolerate. Probably in any setting he would be a workaholic. The others had different priorities and values and set themselves different workloads. All would be successful doctors but would not form a successful partnership.

responsibilities. However, a partnership of relaxed people in touch with their social side may get on well, and a partnership of keen innovators dedicated to patient care may also work (*see* Example 24). Join the wrong sort of partnership, however, and it will be a disaster.

Example 24
When Doctor N (see Example 21) joined her new practice she realised that the workload would be high, although the financial rewards would also be high. She was used to a high workload, having worked for two years in a very busy obstetrics and gynaecology department before turning to general practice, and she enjoyed a challenge. She therefore coped well in her new practice.

Use the non-judgemental value rating scale (*see* Figure 5.1) to consider your own position. Then compare it with your partners'. If you all hold absolutely identical views the practice may become stereotyped, whereas if there is a significant difference, the resulting 'creative tension' will lead to conflict, which paralyses a practice. You can 'plot' your position on the triangle to compare with others. (*See also* Box 5.1.)

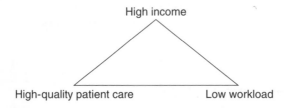

Figure 5.1 The non-judgemental value rating scales (NJVRS).

Box 5.1: NJVRS: balancing income, workload and quality of care

A doctor's duty is to do everything they possibly can for patients	A doctor's first duty is to preserve his own sanity by not overworking
I need to earn as much as possible to achieve a good lifestyle	I want to provide excellent clinical care, even if this lowers profit margins
There are other things in life apart from work and money. Who cares if I'm in debt as long as I'm happy	Money makes the world go round, chum

Number of sessions

You can obtain a rather more detailed idea of workload by considering how many surgeries per week you want or need to do. Then, add on the time that will be needed for administrative and management work, and outside commitments. The nominal 26 hours per week of the full-time principal can very easily become a real 60-hour week.

You will need to offer enough appointments to see your patients, of course. The national average consultation rate is about 3.5 appointments per patient per year, but higher (about 5.5 or more) in inner city areas, and where appointment length is shorter. You can calculate the number of surgery sessions per week needed by using the following formula:

$$\frac{\text{Consultation rate} \times \text{Practice population}}{\text{No. of consultations/hour} \times 52 \text{ weeks} \times \text{Length of surgery}} = \text{No. surgeries/week}$$

Length of appointments offered may determine workload. Shorter appointments may seem to get through the work more quickly, and longer appointments are less stressful for the doctor, improve the quality of care for patients, and reduce the consultation rate per year. Will you aim for 5-, 10- or 15-minute consultations?

How will you allocate special clinic sessions (e.g. baby clinic, minor surgery, diabetic clinic, etc.)? You could each share, perhaps on a rota system, so that everyone keeps up to date, or you may have a special interest partner, who might de-skill those not providing that area of care. Or, you might decide on some other combination arrangements.

Administrative work

- How will you measure the workload of the administration of the practice?
- How will it be shared out (see above)?
- How will profit shares reflect this?

Management work both within the practice (e.g. clinical governance) and outside (e.g. being on the PCG board), can take up a lot of time, and this will probably increase as PCGs become more complex. Make allowances for this in your working week.

Leave

When it comes to leave arrangements you will need to balance the sanity and humanity of partners against the cost of locums (or the increased workload for other partners if you choose to go for an internal cover arrangement). You will need to consider either a practice policy on locum employment to cover leaves, or agree to cover each other's time off.

Refer to the workload non-judgemental rating scales (NJVRS) in Box 5.1 and consider your own position in the triangle shown in Figure 5.2.

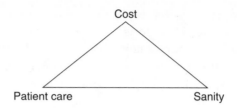

Figure 5.2 The workload triangle.

Remember that locums can cost up to £900 per week, depending on how much locum cover you use, so the more time off you have, the less take-home pay, or the more work you create for your colleagues. For prolonged sick leave, some practices are entitled to locum cost reimbursement from the health authority, depending on the average list size per remaining partner.

The following eight categories of leave are dealt with in our partnership deed. You might wish to consider terms for any or all of these.

1 **Annual leave:** six weeks is common, but remember the cost. Will it be feasible for more than one partner to be away at the same time? Much will depend on the practice size.
2 **Study leave:** you will need some study leave for continued professional development, but do you really want to cover your partner while he enjoys a three-week PGEA course in Portugal, brushing up his golf? Do you want a say in what a partner takes study leave for?
3 **Sick leave:** this is straightforward for short periods, but what about longer sick leave? Will you need individual insurance to cover the costs of this? Will the sick partner have to pay locum costs, or will the practice, and for how long? If the health authority will not pay locum costs you will need to ensure that each partner has his/her own locum expenses policy.
4 **Maternity leave:** you are self-employed, thus not covered by the usual employment rules, although the maternity leave arrangement must not be worse than an equivalent sick leave arrangement for a male partner. (It seems very strange to me that maternity leave should be compared to sick leave, but this is employment law.) Ensure that you have an agreement that is acceptable to you.

5 **Paternity leave:** very trendy, but necessary, believe me – I speak
   as a father of five. How long will you give a new dad? In our
   deed, we allow four weeks, but I think this is unusual.
   Remember, you may have completed your family but the newly
   married partner with strong views on contraception may take a
   special interest in this clause.
6 **Sabbatical leave:** absences for three months or more can cause
   major practice disruption so how often do you want partners
   to be away for long periods, and who will fund it? Sabb-
   aticals are very attractive to the partner taking them, who
   may see this as a way to revive a tired career and come back
   refreshed.
7 **Compassionate leave:** you cannot in all humanity make hard
   and fast rules about compassionate leave, but rough guides and
   examples in the deed may give you a framework on which to
   base decisions, should the need ever arise.
8 **Religious observance leave:** will you make special provision for
   pious members of the practice to observe the major holy days of
   their tradition? Is this fair to the godless partners? We have an
   agreement that partners should not be asked to be on call on a
   major holy day of their tradition, other than in exceptional
   circumstances.

Another type of leave considered is **adoption leave**, equivalent to
maternity leave. This is not in our partnership deed but you may
wish to think about it.

Out-of-hours work

This is another trade-off between sanity, money and patient care.
Again consider the NJVRS shown in Figure 5.3.
   Out-of-hours work can be very stressful, but some doctors feel
they ought to provide this service, because no one will do the job for
their patients as well as they can. Doing all your own cover all the
time will generate good income, but even on a shared rota system it
is very hard work. You can, however, be fairly sure of the quality

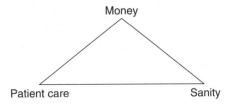

Figure 5.3 The out-of-hours workload triangle.

of care offered. So, some practices do all their own on-call work and, of course, in some areas this is the only option.

Being part of a cooperative is a popular option but can be expensive. Depending on how the cooperative works you may be able to recover the cost or even generate profit by working extra shifts if it allows this. Some partners may wish to do more cooperative work than others to meet personal financial needs. You may feel that patient care can be a little variable but it still tends to be appropriate because members of the cooperative have a vested interest in providing care which their colleagues will approve of.

Using a deputising service can be cheap or costly depending on the arrangement negotiated. Visit rates tend to be higher than for cooperatives and it may be harder to monitor the quality of care of deputies. With a deputy, the partner is responsible for the deputy's actions on issues concerning terms and conditions of service (and a situation could arise where there is a service committee hearing because of a deputy's failing). However, in a cooperative the doctor (provided that he is a principal) is responsible for him/herself. On negligence issues, all doctors are responsible for themselves. Using a deputising service will mean that you do not have to take a turn on the cooperative rota, but again this does depend on the particular cooperative.

Ultimately, the debate between cooperatives and deputising services is really about philosophy rather than sharp differences in service provision, as there is so much variation between cooperatives. A deputising service is really about providing a pragmatic solution to a practice's on-call work at reasonable cost and quality. Cooperatives appear to have a vision of local practices working together, providing innovative solutions to on-call work, and changing the expectations of doctors and patients. Since the development of the cooperative, there has been an enormous change in the entire out-of-hours arena, and it seems likely that in the future, on-call services will change again, perhaps with more co-ordination between general practitioners, accident and emergency departments, social services, and night nursing services.

6

Working policies

There are many areas in practice work which can lead to conflict. In this chapter I have highlighted a few of the issues that might cause problems, and invite you to think about and discuss them before disagreement leads to tension.

Clinical governance within the practice

- How will you keep well informed on the quality of clinical care in the practice?
- Will one partner have a lead responsibility or are all partners equally responsible?
- Who will lead on audit and what audit arrangements will you have?
- What about prescribing costs, complaints or service developments?

These are uncharted areas, but a clinical governance lead for the practice will be needed. This will become a major area of management responsibility, and could be quite a sensitive issue within the practice, because just as all drivers see themselves as average or above-average ability, no one sees themselves as being an under-performing doctor. The clinical governance lead will need to try to create a culture of development and continual learning in the practice, as well as honest appraisal and feedback. All very easy then!

Professional education

You have decided about study leave, but will you make requirements that your partners attend courses, or demonstrate competencies, or perhaps share their learning portfolio.

- How will you ensure that people take time to learn and develop?
- Do you want an appraisal system for doctors, as well as for staff, and if so what type of system?
- How will you ensure that remedial action for problems, service developments and professional development are all facilitated and balanced?

Clinical policies

- Do you want to develop clinical policies to which you all agree (which takes a lot of time and effort)?
- Will you prefer to protect clinical freedom?
- Can you all agree to work in the same way on some issues?
- How will you deal with deviation from the policy? (*See* Box 6.1.)

Box 6.1: NJVRS: tolerating different clinical approaches

There are right and wrong ways of practising medicine so we need as many protocols as possible to reduce variability between doctors

Something as diverse as distress in human beings needs a variety of responses. There are many ways to get to the same end

---

Practice area

The larger the practice area the lower the turnover rate, but home visiting may become a problem. You can keep visit rates down by ringing patients before each visit, but different doctors may have different views on visiting patients at home which might be a source of conflict. Some partners may wish to hang on to long-term patients who move away (*see* Example 25).

Example 25

In a three-doctor practice there had been a tradition of hanging on to patients who moved a short distance from the practice area if they were well known to the doctor. However, two partners did not feel comfortable challenging patients on unreasonable requests and gradually it was found that patients were being allowed to stay on the list when they had moved several miles away. The third partner could tolerate this for a while because she would have been outvoted in a confrontation, but matters came to a head when the cooperative refused to provide cover for some of these patients. Eventually, they agreed to restrict the boundaries. However, perhaps an open discussion about the real issues at an earlier stage may have prevented the problem. They could perhaps have worked out an easier way of telling patients to find new doctors by involving the practice manager, or sticking to a strict rule, rather than trying to defend a wavy line.

In-hours emergency policy

Another key area of clinical policy is how to deal with the emergency that arises during surgery hours. Will there be one doctor delegated to see all emergencies for each day on a rota basis, or will they be fitted in to see their usual doctor? If you operate personal lists and feel continuity is important you may go for the latter option, but it can be disruptive.

7

Final thought

Take care with your choices about partnership. Spend time thinking, discussing and exploring. There is no rush, and there is plenty of locum work for vocationally trained general practitioners. Consider the non-partnership options that are open to you, particularly the newer salaried options. But, above all, try not to let all this get in the way of the central joy of general practice which is the consultation, and the human interactions which it contains.

Appendix

List of main possible sources of practice income and expense, including non-GMS work.

Income

Basic practice allowance
Seniority
Postgraduate education
    allowance
Assistant allowance
Out-of-hours allowance

Capitation fees
Deprivation fees
New registration fee
Child health surveillance fees

Item of service fees
  out-of-hours consultation
  maternity
  contraception
  immunisations
  temporary resident
  immediately necessary
    treatment
  emergency treatment

Targets
  cervical smear
  childhood immunisation

Minor surgery

Health promotion annual fee
Chronic disease management
    fee
  diabetes
  asthma

Reimbursements
  rent and rates
  staff salaries (usually 70%)
  staff training costs
  computer costs
Improvement grants
Special grants

Non-core work (depends on
    PCG agreements)

nursing home
anti-coagulation clinic
drug abuse work
HRT implants
antirheumatics

Hospital sessions (e.g. clinical
assistant)
Work for cooperative

PCG work
Private medicals, certificates,
reports and forms

Benefits Agency work
Police surgeon
Prison work
Occupational health
Work for charitable and
voluntary organisations

Education, lecturing, course
organising etc.
SIFTR (medical student
teaching)
Training grant GPRs

Expenses

Drugs and instruments
Locum and cooperative fees
NHS levies (money deducted to
support the LMC)

Premises expenses
rent and rates
heat and light
insurance
repairs

Staff expenses
salaries and NI
training
recruitment
catering

Office expenses

Bank costs
Legal costs
Accountants costs
Cleaning costs

GPR, general practice research; HRT, hormone replacement therapy; LMC, Local Medical Committee; NI, National Insurance; PCG, Primary Care Group; SIFTR, Service Increment for Teaching and Research.

Index

accountants 37–8
accounts 37–8
  inspection by interviewees 36–7
administrative work 44
administrators 19–20
adoption leave 46
annual leave 45
appointments
  length of 44
  number of 43–4
assessment periods 24
assistantships 21–2

banking policy 37–8
Belbin's group roles 8

Cabinet structure 14
car expenditure 34
clinical governance within practice
  49–50
clinical policies 50
clinics 44
community trust property 30
compassionate leave 46
compulsory expulsion 25–6
conflict 42
  dealing with 12
  in 'senior partner as executive'
    model 14
  sources of 49–51

clinical governance within
    practice 49–50
clinical policies 50
in-house emergency policy 51
practice area 51
professional education 50
cooperatives 3, 9, 47–8
core values 1–3
  of practice 3–5
corporate culture 3
course fees 34
course organisers 33

debts, responsibility for 17, 38
decision making 17–18
  'democracy and shared
    responsibility' model 14–15
  joint responsibility for 16–17
  'senior partner as executive
    model' 13–14
  total democratic model 16
  see also management teams
democracy and shared responsibility
  model 14–15
  total democratic model 16
deputising services 47

education 50
  training practice status 5
emergency policy 51

employment law issues 16–17
   maternity leave and 45
executive, senior partner as 13–14
expenses 56
   pooling of 34
expulsion, compulsory 25–6

financial issues 31–9
   accounts 37–8
   banking policy 37–8
   goodwill, sale of 35–6
   outside work, attitudes toward
      32–3
   partnership shares 34–5
   pooling expenses 34
   pooling income 31–2
   private patients 38–9
   showing accounts to interviewees
      36–7
financial risk 28, 29

General Medical Council (GMC)
   registration fees 34
general practice registrar (GPR) 5
goodwill, sale of 35–6
groupthink 1, 4
   danger of 4

health authority
   larger practices and 9
   notional rent payments 27–8, 29,
      30

identity, of practice 3–5
in-house emergency policy 51
income
   from outside appointments 32–3
   pooling of 31–2
   sources of 55–6
interviewees, inspection of accounts
   36–7
investment in premises 27–8

job-sharing 20–1

larger practices 9–10

leased premises 29–30, 31
leave 44–6
legal responsibilities 16–17
linked small practices 10–11
list size 41
loans for premises 27–8
Local Medical Committees (LMCs)
   35
locums, cost of 44–5

majority vote 17
management teams
   administrative work 44
   Belbin's group roles 8
   within partnership 15
   see also decision making
managers 18–20
maternity leave 45
minor surgery 23–4
   income from 32
moral stance 1–3
mutual assessment periods 24

negligence issues 47
non-judgemental value rating scales
   (NJVRS) viii, 42–7
notional rent payments 27–8

on-call work 46–8
out-of-hours work 46–8
outside appointments 32–3
owned premises 27–9

parity, progression to 24–5, 35
part-time working 20–1
partnership vii–ix
   dynamics between partners 12–13
      democracy and shared
         responsibility 14–15
      management team within
         partnership 15
      senior partner as executive 13–
         14
      total democratic model 16
   number of partners 9–12
      larger practices 9–10

small practices   11–12
small practices linked   10–11
partnership shares   34–5
salaried partners   22–3
team roles   7–8
Partnership Act (1890)   viii
partnership deed   vii–viii
paternity leave   46
patients
allocation of   23–4
appointments
length of   44
number of   43–4
list size   41
private patients   27–8, 38–9
personal core values   1–3
personal lists   23–4
police surgeons   33
pooling of expenses   34
pooling of income   31–2
Postgraduate Education Allowance
(PGEA)   32
practice administrator   19–20
practice area   51
practice debts, responsibility for   17,
38
practice manager   18–20
practices
clinical governance   49–50
identity   3–5
number of partners   9–12
larger practices   9–10
small practices   11–12
small practices linked   10–11
primary care group (PCG)
involvement   6
training practice status   5
types of   3, 4
see also partnership
premises
leasing of   29–30, 31
owning of   27–9
rent for community trust property
30
primary care group (PCG)
involvement   6

larger practices   9
workload and   9, 44
prior shares   31–2
private patients   38–9
notional rent payments and   27–8
professional education   50
professional memberships   34
professional stance   1–3
profit-sharing ratios   31–2, 34–5
progression to parity   24–5, 35
psychological profiling   7

qualified majority vote   17

Red Book   19, 29
religious observance leave   46
rent and rates payments   27–8
rent for community trust property   30
responsibility
for decision making   16–17
for practice debts   17, 38
legal responsibilities   16–17
shared responsibility model   14–15
restricted covenant clauses   25

sabbatical leave   46
salaried partners   22–3
sale of goodwill   35–6
senior partner as executive model
13–14
seniority payments   32
sessions, number of   43–4
shared responsibility model   14–15
sick leave   45
single-handed practices   11
small practices   11–12
linked small practices   10–11
special clinics   44
stereotypes   3, 42
study leave   45
superpractices   9
surgery sessions, number of   43–4

tax liability   38
team roles   7–8
total democratic model   16
training practice status   5

true managers   18–19

unanimous vote   17

values   1–3
  of practice   3–5
vehicle expenditure   34

workload   41–2
  administrative work   44
  leave   44–6
  number of sessions   43–4
  out-of-hours work   46–8
  primary care group (PCG)
    involvement and   6